More Than a Pretty Face

The True Story of my life
10 years after Weight Loss Surgery

Kelsey Payumo

Table of Contents

HELLO & WELCOME!

Hello and WELCOME! My name is Kelsey and I had Gastric Bypass weight loss surgery 10 years ago. I lost 256 pounds, had a baby, regained 90+ pounds, got divorced, moved across the country, lost my regain, and learned to love myself through it all.

I wanted to share my story with YOU!

Why you? Because if you are like me and you struggle with life after WLS - it's easy to feel lost and helpless. Whets hard is finding the motivation to keep going and keep pushing towards your goals. It's also hard when you feel like you're alone. YOU ARE NOT ALONE and you are going to be okay.

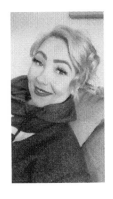

In this book, I go through my story, and the different life events I found myself facing in the last 10 years. Some of it gets brutally honest, especially when talking about WHY I had Weight Loss Surgery, and How I Lost My Regain. But regardless, it's a testimony to the strength each of us has within; we sometimes just need a little push to get it to come out.

So let's get started: Here is my story.

MY STORY - WHY I HAD GASTRIC BYPASS AND WHAT HAPPENED NEXT

Here is my story of weight loss surgery – I had gastric bypass in 2008. I lost a total of 256 pounds and took my life back. It's written blog style.

Hi everyone, anyone, no one, you:

Where should I start? Age 16 when I first noticed I wasn't really the same size as all the other girls? Age 17 when I didn't make the volleyball team because I was viewed as fat which somehow equaled bad? Age 21 when I couldn't find any pants that fit me anywhere in the entire mall?

All of my conscious adult life, I've been fat. Unapologetically so. So much so that if you made some sort of comment about it, I'd turn it around into a joke and most often enough to make you blush. I've never been the girl with the sad story who cried at night because I wasn't a size 2. I've never been the girl who never had a boyfriend because my ass was twice the size of the next girl's.

I have been the girl who could come up with the most elaborate excuse as to why I'm about to eat this, or why I'd ate that and that yesterday. I've also been the girl who centered her entire life around food and the process of consuming it.

It ends today.

Dr. Chang (who you will get to know more as this blog progresses) said something to me on Wednesday that absolutely struck me as the most truth since blonde hair doesn't suit my skin colour: Nothing Tastes as Good as Thin.

Lets take a moment to drink that in.

Nothing Tastes as Good as Thin.

I know what you're thinking, well some of you; "what is this girl going on about, I love my body no matter what and no one should tell me I have to be thin to be happy." Honey, I've been there. Sitting here at my computer in size 26-28 yoga pants, I am telling you, I have been there as recently as yesterday. There is nothing wrong with self love. There is absolutely nothing wrong with being self confident. There is definately nothing wrong with strutting your stuff like the Queen you are. But what is wrong is looking into the mirror with such undying affection that it causes your common sense to go unheard. It is wrong to pull on your size 28 pants and suck in to button them up and see your belly snug like a bug in a rug. There is something wrong when you look at your measurements with a blind eye to the fact that you are as big around as you are tall.

When I got up this morning, brushing my teeth and looking into the mirror, I was bombarded with thoughts and questions. Do I think I'll live to see 50? No. Do I think I'll live to see babies of my babies? No. When I really get honest with myself, do I even see my own babies? No. But do I think I'm beautiful? Yes.

This is where the past year has caught up to me. For the past year, I've been trying to lose weight. Trying is maybe too strong of a word. I've been conscious of the idea of trying to lose weight. Trying to walk the very thin rope of health while underneath me, happiness is rooting for me to fall. I've been happy being fat. I've been happy going out to eat every night, eating whatever I wanted without consequence. While I've been so happy, my body has been crying out for some help. Migraines, insomnia, stomach aches, sore ankles, aching knees, have all been signs my body is unhappy. But my old friend Tylenol was there to soothe the pain. Until February 8th, 2008. On this day, I was hit with a pain that no medicine could ease. A pain no amount of prayer, sleep nor distraction could even come close to erasing. That was the day my body finally gave up and took from me the only thing in the world I have ever truly wanted: a baby. Even now, 8 months later, it still hurts. Although this wasn't the first time by body had done this to me; it was made obvious to me what my body was saying this time:

"Kelsey, please get help"

After the physical trauma subsided a bit, and the emotional eating wore it's self out, I finally got the nerve to go in and see the woman who had previously told me that I was too fat to ever get pregnant. In that little windowless office I cried like a baby being hugged by a woman who I had hated. I asked her why so many times. I reminded her that I had no diagnosed issues surrounding my weight. I pleaded with her to help me. I was doing the unthinkable. I was asking her to help me find a way to lose weight.

(For some of you reading this, this might be getting a bit too personal, and I do apologize but I feel it necessary for myself to have the entire process documented, including the lead up and my reasons why.)

Once she managed to calm me down and we were able to talk freely she suggested that I look into surgical weight loss. The thought has always been in the back of my head but never more than I passing fancy. I always thought "I don't need the easy way out – if I wanted to lose weight, I could." Well quite obviously I couldn't. We talked and talked. She knew of my constant dieting and then binging. She knew of the pills upon pills upon shakes upon programs for weight loss. What she was seeing now though was new: desperation. She and I both knew that losing another baby because I can't say no to eating two full portions of pasta was going to kill me. So she made the first move in my journey and put together a referal.

The next few steps of this I will just bulletin point:

> Doctor sends in referal
> Tricare refers a hospital 8 hours away
> I find someone closer who takes Tricare
> I wait 2 months for an appointment
> I go in to be told that I'm actually too fat for weight loss surgery (what in the hell?)
> I kinda give up
> I meet Sue.

Sue. I can't even begin to describe how much I owe to Sue. Sue and I met at Curves. She's a petite lady who just actually had her 60th birthday but doesn't really look a day over 40. She's always had a quick smile and a laugh to share. I honestly didn't know Sue that well until I was working out a Curves one day, chit chatting with Lee – one of the trainers and talking about how I couldn't believe this doctor in the city told me I was too fat for medical weight loss. Lee mentioned that Sue had gastric bypass and if I'd like it if she gave Sue my number and we could talk. At this point, I was convinced I only wanted the Lap Band (I will explain the procedures more in depth shortly). Sue called me and we talked and she mentioned that her doctor had a practice only one hour from here and that it was one of only two centre's of excellence in the country. My excitement kinda started to creep back in. She gave me his name and told me to call and see if they took his insurance. Getting up the nerve to call was something I had to work on, after being told I was too fat, I was so scared of that rejection again. The nicest woman answered the phone and told me that no, they didn't take Tricare but that his partner who just opened his own practice did and she gave me that number. So I called them and they set me up an appointment right away. About 2 weeks later I met Dr. Chang.

Let's talk about Dr. Chang for a bit. Not only is he extremely cute but he's very to the point. He doesn't pussy foot around the issues. When I walked into his office at 327 pounds he said "we can do this, but you're going to have to help me." I was scared. I was so scared he was going to say, lose 100 pounds and we'll talk – because if I could lose 100 pounds on my own, I wouldn't be in there right? And he ACTUALLY said that. He realized that I've been on every diet under the sun and that I was coming to him to do something I couldn't do alone.

Leaving Dr. Chang's office that day, I felt a new sense of understanding and also like a changed woman. I understood that my health didn't have to come second anymore. That he and I together could conquer this disease of Obesity.

From the moment I met Sue, she invited me to start going to her weight loss surgery support group. Pouch Pals was a scary thing to commit to. The first meeting, I walked into a room of super models. Well, they aren't, but many of them could be. Skinny and tanned, gorgeous people sitting in a circle around the room. Paul – our moderator – was there and greeting everyone telling them how good they look. I initially kinda figured we had walked in on an ex cheerleaders meeting. I sat down nervously amongst the other 50 people, beside Sue and was silent. Which for those of you that know me, know that's a rare occasion.

We started with Mia. Mia is an absolutely stunning Mexican girl. She started like an AA meeting with a twist, "Hi, I'm Mia and I've lost 202 pounds." I was SHOCKED. What? This girl could never have had 200 pounds on her total! let alone on top of the probably 103 she weighs now. She passed around her photo album and I nearly fell out of my chair. There was the same face, I can see those eyes, and those lips on the girl in front of me...but the bulk around her was astounding. As I flipped the pages, I found that I had been holding my breath. It was truly amazing. As we went around the room introducing ourselves, it was incredible to hear how everyone had lost more than 100 pounds – all thanks to Dr. Chang and Sue's doctor, Dr. McDaniel. When we got to Sue, she proudly stated she had lost 206 pounds. I was shocked again. I knew from that first night on that I too could have this type of success story. I could be a loser.

Fast forward to this Wednesday. One month after meeting Dr. Chang for the first time. I've lost 16 pounds since we met. I've been to see his therapist to make sure my mind was right. I've been to his diet class on how to eat after surgery. He says those magic words "we're ready for surgery." So Amanda, his amazing assistant, puts in my referral for the surgery to Tricare. Fast forward to checking the Tricare website probably every 5 mins until Friday morning. Instead of the P for pending I see an A for approved. I nearly burst.

I am approved. OH MY GOD. I am approved. I AM APPROVED!

That is all for today, but my story will continue later when I find some pictures to show you guys about the procedure, about myself, about my doctor and my friends and my family.

Today is the first day of the rest of my life.

Nothing tastes as good as thin.
Nothing.

Installment #2.

I hate being woken up in the morning. Especially by the phone. My phone rang and as soon as I answered it, it died so I had to run to the other room and see who was calling before it went on speaker.

me: "Hello?"
Amanda: "Hi Kelsey, this is Amanda from Dr. Chang's office, how are you?"
me groggily: "I'm good Amanda, how are you?"
Amanda: "Great, I was just calling to set up your surgery date, when would you like to have surgery?"
me awake: "5 years ago"
Amanda: "*laughing* okay well, you're in for your preop tomorrow, how does Thursday sound for surgery?"
me very awake now: "that sounds fantastic"

Thursday, September 25th, 2008 my life will change forever. With a very few scars I will remember that day as the day I no longer let food dominate my life. I will remember that even though the road was hard, that was the day I took back control.

<u>Installment #3.</u>

Pre-Op

I don't really get that scared that easily. But walking into the hospital today for my preop all alone was scary. I know I can do this, I know I'm going to be okay but I'm scared. I have very little support as it stands right now from family – they are simply too far away. I have my WLS support group who are awesome and my girls from work who are amazing but I feel so very very alone. I cried twice on my drive home from the hospital today. First because I'm scared and second because I'm alone. But this was my choice to be very far from my family who are busy with their own lives, I know I can't expect them to drop everything and come to me. I'd give anything to have someone here with me.

I know that waking up in the recovery room is going to hit home just how alone I really am but when it comes down to it, I know that I am strong enough to face this and any other challenge life throws at me. I know I can do this.

I know I sound depressed today, I'm just really tired, anxious, nervous and a little disappointed. Plus being on a water diet for the next week is starting to wear on me after the first day. But I have to remind myself that all of this is worth it. Nothing tastes as good as thin.

So I go back Thursday morning, Lily is driving me there, at 4am we will leave my house. The beginning of my brand new life. I can't wait.

Installment #4.

The Day Before

Waking up this morning I felt a little different. I little more resolved, a little less scared and alot more hungry. When I got to the doctor's office (for my overseas screening female testing thingy) and they weighed me, I was shocked to see I lost 6 pounds...in 24 HOURS!!?!? I guess perhaps the water diet does really work eh? *laugh* Dr. Chang will be happy to see that he will have a little more room to work tomorrow I'm sure.

Home Again, Flanagan

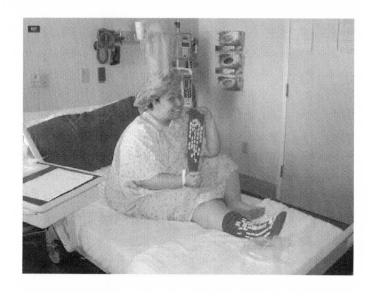

Ya, I don't know where that saying came from either, except that my Mum used to say it every time we got home from somewhere. It was as vital as saying in our car growing up as "put your clicks on or this is where the parade was. *laugh* Childhood memories are great. So. I'm home. Whew. I'm home and alive. Really, the best two things I could wish for. First of all, I'd like to send love and thanks and hugs and chocolate to my wonderful Nurses at 6th South. For them to wait on me hand and foot, even when I was difficult was a testimony to amazing. You ladies rock. Seriously.

To Dr. Chang. Thank you are two words that get the general meaning of what I want to say to you, although they are only a drop in the barrel. I am forever to remember you as the man who saved my life.

So, Thursday, Lily picked me up at 5am and we drove to Victoria. It was early, although I barely slept, too anxious. We arrive at the hospital. We go upstairs to the 6th floor – I felt like I had walked onto the set of House. There were hardwood floors as far as the eye could see. And not that fakiehardwood. Hardwood like my parent's house (minus the lines) and even hardwood designs in the hallways. There was soft lighting on the Nurses' Station who when the elevator opened they all turned and smiled at me at the same time. I was completely overwhelmed. I was then taken to my private room which also had hardwood. It also had a beautiful rocking chair, a day bed, my bed, a huge bathroom and marble counters around the sink.

I can't make this up guys! It also showed a gorgeous view of the park outside the hospital as I was on the 6th floor. I cannot get over the beauty and hospitality of this place. I definitely didn't feel like I was in a hospital. So about 10 mins after I came in, my wonderful Nurse came down with a computer on a cart and asked me a bazillion questions, took my vitals, weighed me (I was down 8 pounds in the two days previous) and handed me my operation gown and socks. Now, for those of you who have never been fat I have something to share: Hospital gowns, never, ever, ever fit.

They are always left gaping. Okay so I'm worried, I don't want to sit around for 2 hours getting ready for surgery showing everyone my naked body – the front view too! But I do as she asks and put it on. I'm shocked when it fits. In fact, I could wrap it around myself 3 times! Finally, somewhere that knew how to deal with us. Finally.

Over the course of the next three days I would hear various staff from the hospital say how 6th south got special treatment and this floor was not only prettier but also that the staff here was trained specifically to treat you like you were the Queen of England. Boy did I luck out. God Bless Texas (at least in this area). Next I get shots, she's telling me what they are for and I finish her sentences. I have researched every single part of this procedure. I'm not one to go in blind. I get the heparin in my belly to prevent blood clots and something stoma behind my ear in patch form to help with the nausea later. I also get an IV with a PCMpump. A PCM for those of you that don't know is a Pain Control Machine. It allows me to administer my morphine by the click of a pump that is attached to my IV. I was thinking "finally, no more having to hit the call button when I'm in agony." Boy was I wrong. After she left, my OR nurse comes in. She asks me to get on the table/bed and covers me in warm heated blankets. MMMgood.

At this point, I was biting back tears saying goodbye to Lily who sat with me there for 2 hours and got up at 4am to drive me. As I was wheeling down the hallway, Miss Nanette (the head of that department) called to me by name and wished me luck and said she'd stop by in a few hours. She called me by NAME. I felt like I was a person and not some number going through there. So down we go in the elevator, we pass by rooms and rooms of stainless steel equipment and my nervousness grows with each step.

Finally I'm rolled into the waiting room for surgery. A beautiful OR assistant comes over, introduces herself and starts me a different IV since mine had seemed to stop working (this happened three times over the course of the three days, I have bad disappearing veins apparently). She was so gentle it didn't hurt a bit. The Anesthesiologist (I can't spell to save my life sorry) comes in and says "Hi Kelsey, are you ready for your cocktail?" This breaks my tension and nervousness right up and I laugh and say, "please". He gives me something to relax and then I see the man of the hour. Dr. Chang walks in scrubs and asks how I'm feeling. I just smile as again I'm biting back tears, which he can tell and says everything looks great and "wow great job on the extra eight pounds, you've given me so much room to work this is going to go great!" which again helped ease the anxiety. At this point, things get pretty fuzzy. The clock on the wall is directly in front of me and I watch the seconds tick past and finally I'm moving. We go into the operating room and I see the tools, the cameras, and about 10 people smiling. I scoot over onto that table and lay back, as the anesthesia takes hold I remember saying, "please don't let me wake up during this okay" and I'm out.

Fast forward three hours. I wake up in recovery. I don't remember lot except for the male nurse over me with a United States Marine Corp layette around his neck saying "miss, please stop crying, we're going to give you something for the pain." I don't remember the pain but if I woke up crying, I guess there must have been some. The next thing I remember is waking up again in my room with 3 nurses in there telling me to sit up a little so they can put a pillow behind my back and take my blood pressure. Dr. Chang comes in and gives me what looks like a picture of intestines, says the surgery went perfectly and that he'd see me later and I'm out again.

The next time I wake up, I'm feeling the pain so I hit my PCM for the morphine. Probably every 20 minutes I hit the machine for more. It's weird to describe now but I remember telling my nurses that on the 1-10 scale, my pain was hovering around 8-9. The morphine keeps knocking me out but each time I wake up, I have to pee. SO the nurse helps me up and out of my oxygen tube, my leg compression things (which are these things that they put around your calves that blow up and then deflate and are heated so you don't get blood clots) and when I finally get into the bathroom, I'm nearly in tears because no matter how long I sit there, I cannot pee. I remember asking the nurse to please call my parents because they must be worried and strangely enough I only can remember my Dad's cell phone number. Back into the bed machines are constantly beeping and waking me up. I feel like I can get no rest. More morphine. Pretty soon my nurse is distressed. Each time I fall asleep, my oxygen level falls drastically and causes that machine to alert and thus I'm not getting any sleep. Pretty soon I'm extremely nauseous and shortly after that the migraine hits home. I can't open my eyes, the morphine has stopped working, I'm in absolute agony. I lay there crying, trying not to because it makes the migraine worse. My nurses are unsure what to do. Finally they realize that I'm having a reaction to the morphine. Because I'm pumped full of the stuff by that point, they want me to get up and walk the halls to help the gas pain (when they do my bypass laproscopically, they blow your belly up with Co2 gas which causes pain if it doesn't get released and unfortunately mine was not coming out except in occasional hiccups.) So up I get and walk, my belly is hurting, my head is hurting more and I feel like I'm about to vomit at any second only there is nothing to vomit so it's heaving. I do one lap and collapse on the bed. I'm exhausted. The nurses come in yet again and give me an oral pain medicine which thankfully does the trick quickly but by this point it is 7am and I've had a sleepless night.

Fast forward to the next day at 2pm. I finally wake up feeling rested but still in pain in my belly. This is mostly gas pain and not surgery pain since you can't really feel your stomach. They urge me to walk so I walk but the gas will not work itself out. I get up every two hours and do 2 laps around my floor. The walking feels good and when I get back into bed, I just fall right back asleep. When I am awake I'm using this breathing device that helps my lungs stay strong and also sipping on water. One sip makes me feel full quickly so it's a slow process. I was overjoyed the afternoon that they brought in chicken bouillon. Finally something with taste. I measure out my one ounce and sit there sipping it for an hour. One ounce of liquid in one hour. It was insane. But I felt good. The pain was still there but it was manageable with the oral pills.

Fast forward to Saturday. I wake up feeling sparky pain under my rips. The gas bubbles are having a party and then suiciding on my rips. Good, finally getting out of my belly. The pain is still there but I'm dealing. I can finally pee too! A miracle. X-ray comes in to do my upper GI, to be sure that there are no leaks in my pouch and small intestine around the internal incision sites. So a lovely woman named Petunia comes and wheels me down into the "freezer". It was hellaciously cold in there. Thankfully I didn't have to wait long and I get taken into the X-ray room. They make me drink this liquid they say tastes like Kerosene. DISGUSTING. I nearly vomited right there. Then I stood up against the x-ray machine and watched this fluid go through my new stomach (called the pouch) and into my small intestine. I wasn't entirely sure what I was looking at but they took a bunch of pictures and I was sent back upstairs. A few hours later, the on call surgeon came in to tell me that I needed to have another upper GI x-ray. He said there was potentially a problem so he wanted to look again. Down I go, more disgusting liquids and this time 3 people in there watching it go through. They determine that nothing is indeed wrong and I'm sent back upstairs with a pouch so full I thought I might puke on the way up. My pouch only holds two teaspoons of liquid at this point and drinking like 6 ounces of this nasty stuff was really too much.

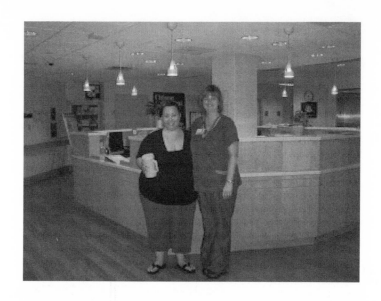

Fast forward to discharge time. Sara and Lily arrive and its home again time. Whew. I made it. I was feeling good and the drive home was nice. We had a 4 hour run around at Walgreen's over my meds but in the end Donna the nursing supervisor at the hospital came through and got me what I needed. And finally around 9pm that night, I was home, snug as a bug in a rug in my own bed.

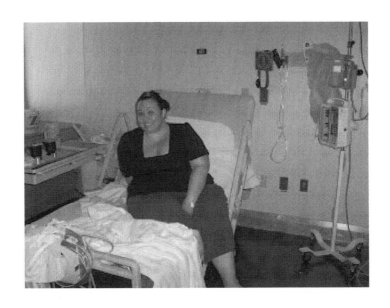

So that's my surgery story. Boy it was long. Took me nearly a week to write it all out. Through it all Dr. Chang has been my #1 supporter. He called me at 9:40pm on Saturday night after I was worried I couldn't swallow the large pain pills I was prescribed. He reassured me I would be okay and said to call him anytime, no matter what time, no matter for what. He really is the best doctor I've ever encountered. Ever. More to come soon lovelies.

Installment #6.

Day 1-7 – Great! Day 8 – not so great!

I was doing fine, even great up until last night. They have me on Darvocet for the pain and the pills are pretty big. Given that the entrance to my pouch from my throat is only the size of the end of a pencil, things have to be really small to fit through. Well I've been cutting up the pills into thirds and unfortunately last night, one got stuck in the opening. It was more scary than anything but after a two am crying phone call to my doctor, he said to sip warm liquids until it passes. I don't think it has passed yet though. I also think I've not been drinking enough water. I'm supposed to get down 70oz per day and so far I've managed 30oz and I'm starting to feel the effects, really weak and migraine headaches, which I can't take anything for because my pouch opening is blocked. So I've been crushing the darvocet and mixing well with water and sipping on that. Disgusting but migraines are nothing to fool with. Other than that, things are pretty good. I've graduated to 1oz (think shot glass) meals of 99% fat free cream soups over 30 mins (hahah I eat with a baby spoon again!) and boy, potato soup yesterday was an incredible treat for me. Having the taste of real food in your mouth rather than milk or water was almost overwhelming.

I have still had the problem with the gas. It just won't come out but finally I had my first bowel movement in a week so I hope the gas is next in line. I don't feel as bloated anymore but when I sleep – my insides still feel sore. So things are slowly moving along.

I see Dr. Chang on Thursday so he will tell me how much weight I've lost since then. I hope it's alot. hahah. They say don't weigh for the first two weeks because as your body heals, it retains more water and will give you a false understanding, like in the hospital I gained 5 pounds of water weight. After that, they say to weigh once a week, most of the ladies in my support group though weigh every day. Obesity isn't just about weight, it's a disease and one that never really goes away. Much like an alcoholic. In order to keep on top of it, I have to be aware of every single thing I put into my body. I'm fairly confident that I will most likely never eat bread again. As much as it pains me to say that because it is something that I can easily overdo. I've always loved breads of any sort and for me, that was my gateway to this disease. But we'll see what the future holds. I'm not craving anything really yet although last night I had an extremely vivid dream of eating pizza. Boy do I love pizza and I hope that one day, I might be able to eat a small piece of whole wheat pizza or something of the like.

It's now 8pm and I'm going to sit down and watch some TV before bed. Most likely CNN to watch Sarah Palin get destroyed in reviews of her on the debate last night. She really makes all women look bad. I'm going to stop saying that I'm from the part of Canada connected to Alaska. Anyway guys. Lots of love from me to you. This road may be hard but nothing tastes as good as thin.

<u>Installment #7.</u>

RIP – my first weight loss since surgery

Today I said goodbye forever to 22 pounds. Today at Dr. Chang's office I made them weigh me twice because I thought it was some sort of mistake. 22 pounds in 13 days. I feel like I'm on the Amazing Race...only instead of seeing parts of the world, I'm seeing parts of myself falling off.

I feel great. Today marked the last day of the liquid diet also! I've graduated to soft foods such as scrambled eggs, refried beans, yogurt and finely sliced deli meats! HORRAY! real food yay! Of course, I can still only eat about a quarter of a cup over 30 mins but you don't even know how good those beans tasted today. Wow. Of course, everything also has to be fat free and sugar free but still...diet food has never tasted so good.

I'm having a rough time getting in enough water which was causing some headaches. But I'm getting that under control now. Having to set a timer on my cell phone reminding me to drink might seem silly but dehydration is no joke.

Pain – there and back again

So Thursday started off normal. I excitedly got up and made an ounce of scrambled eggs, with a bit of fat free cheese. Sat down for 30 mins and ate it. I don't usually like eggs but it felt good to feel my little pouch all warm and full. At lunch, I had one piece of paper thin deli ham and one ounce of finely chopped cantaloupe. By 2pm my belly was feeling a little rumbly but no big deal, first day on real food. By 3pm I was doubled over in my bed crying from pain. It felt like period cramps times a million.

Now when I had gallbladder disease, a gallbladder attack made me lose my mind, I couldn't see, breathe or move. This was worse. I haven't actually had a baby but it felt like what I imagine contractions to feel like. There would be 30 second intervals of no pain and then it would strike suddenly and make me want to just die.

I laid in my bed for about 6 hours, almost in tears, thinking "what have I done?" Finally after some coaxing and realizing that this is not what bypass patients call "dumping" (I'll explain that later) I called my surgeon. Exactly 3 minutes later he returned my call and calmed me down. He said that I needed to drink with all my meals right now because the food was having a hard time passing through my new openings and thus it was balling up and forcing its way through my intestines. He said to take one of my Darvocet and just relax. I followed his advice and sipped hot tea for the rest of the evening. The pain did not stop but it subsided to a mild cramping that at least I could bare with and then fall asleep.

Despite this small set back, I feel great. Friday and today have been fabulous. I'm getting better at drinking my water, and eating slower. It's funny after just a bite and getting that full feeling. It surprises me every time. In other news, today I put on a pair of jeans I haven't been able to wear in almost two years. I thought what the hell, let's give em a go...lo and behold they fit, if not even a bit too big! It seems like a miracle.

Talking to my sister today I discovered I have more readers than I thought. I'd like to say welcome and thank you for taking an interest in my journey. This surgery has and is changing my life. I don't think it's for everyone as the day to day aspects of it are hard (drinking 70 ounces of water, not pooping for 10 days, not being able to have any sugar or any fat, no alcohol etc) but for me, it's truly saved my life. I'm happy to be able to share my story even from thousands of miles away.

I was reading my towns only newspaper (RIP Robson Valley Times) and saw an article on childhood obesity. The editorial was well written and quoted a lot of facts I have seen time and time again when doing research on Obesity. There was a letter back talking about the causes of it. I think the writer meant well but I honestly believe he completely missed the point. Obesity isn't something you get from eating too many French fries. Obesity isn't taught to us by parents who both work and give their children money for takeout. Obesity isn't caused by computer games keeping kids indoors.

Growing up, as most of you know, I was pretty active. I played almost all the school sports, plus figure skating, plus ballet (sometimes) and my Mum always had a wholesome meal plan for us every single day. I remember going to elementary school and seeing my friends with the snack packs and the processed food and I had a real sandwich on whole wheat bread, and usually some sort of real fruit – usually an apple (right Mum?). I was active in high school nearly every single day. I rarely drank – not of out nutrition but fear of the repercussions from my parents finding out. All in all, I was a very healthy kid. But...I was overweight. I don't remember exactly when it started, I think sometime around grade 7. I remember developing far before any of the other girls in my class so I attributed my weight to that. As the years passed, so did the scale. Despite being active and eating relatively well, I was growing more and more overweight each year.

Looking back now I can clearly identify when I was infected with this disease of Obesity. I have always been a social butterfly. I like to make friends and I love conversation. Nearly every great memory I have with friends has involved food in some way. Family dinners at Byrons, Wing Night, Grill Night, lunches at the Great Escape, etc. Food quickly became a means for people to get together. I can't lay the fault completely there though.

I love food. I have always loved food. I love the tastes and smells. It's a wonder I don't love to cook...hahah. As my relationship with food grew into a stepping stone for socializing, I lost sight of portions and quickly ate my way into being one of the most popular girls at my university and morbidly obese. Because I was always the funny cool girl to hang out with, no one ever commented on my weight, because to them, it didn't matter. To me, it never mattered either. Going out to eat was going out with friends with the added benefit of something yummy. Over time I stretched my stomach out so much that it took alot to get me full. Not to mention that after years of figure skating practice only having a 15 min break for dinner, I learned to eat fast. One of my most notable things was that I would eat alot, lay on the floor and whine for someone to please kill me, I'm about to explode.

That is when obesity consumed me. Even if you eat the right stuff (which I'm not saying I always did, me and the carbs had a torrid love affair) you still can suffer from this disease. Even now that I'm losing weight, I will still be susceptible to this disease rearing its ugly head. Obesity is much like alcoholism, it never goes away, you just have to learn how to manage it. Anyway, that was long winded but I hope it gives a bit more insight into my life.

PREGNANCY AFTER WLS

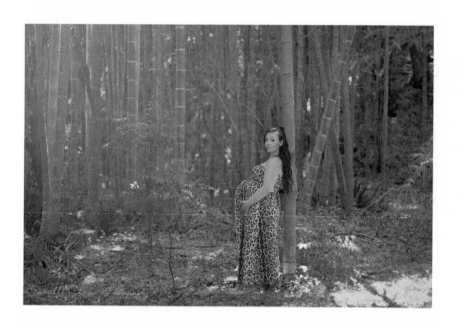

I wanted to take a moment and talk to those of you who are pregnant, trying to become pregnant or hoping to in the future.

I lost 256 pounds and maintained for 3 years. I was doing great, I didn't eat any of the crap and stayed true to my plan.

Life was wonderful. Once I finally decided it was my time to become a Mama – I blessed myself with a very planned pregnancy.

I thought I had all the answers, my Dr was the head of medicine and he was watching me very closely. I was his first bariatric patient who was pregnant and we were learning together. We googled, we called Dr's back in the states (I was living overseas in Japan on a US military base) and we spoke to my surgeon once a week.

Guess what? We messed up big time. We decided that the best thing for me was bed rest, carb reintroduction, and drinking hot tea while I ate to facilitate more consumption. We were both nervous, I was terrified, at that point I had lost 6 pregnancies and this was going to be my last try. He said eat bread, I ate bread. He said eat more potatoes and bananas, and I did.

I ate and I ate, and I was sick, and didn't walk and laid in bed, snacking and watching the seasons change.

I also gained around 55 pounds. My baby boy was born healthy and absolutely perfect in August of 2011.

My Dr was elated that we were able to go through and have a "normal" pregnancy. We thought, "continue to eat like you did while pregnant, you're nursing and your body is healing" and due to my emergency C-Section — I wasn't able to really do much for a long time.

I gained again. The excuses upon excuses upon excuses turned into bad choices, and dumping every other day. I managed to cut the bread but there were so many bariatric websites that preached "EAT IN MODERATION" "ONE BITE CAN'T KILL YOU" "TORTILLAS ARE SAFE" etc etc. I followed one for awhile — gained again. I started the Paleo diet — dumped every time I ate. I did Atkins — gained. I tried everything...because I thought that at 5 years after my RNY — my pouch was broken, I had given away my tool in exchange for this perfect little human in my arms. And I was okay with that.

Enter September 2015. I had been divorced, moved across the country and was sick. Every day I was sick. I decided to start trying to look into revision. I found this site. Susan Maria's book was my bible while I was in Japan – I had no support, my Dr was back in Texas, my medical team on base had never had a bariatric patient. In 2008 you weren't even supposed to get medical clearance from the military to go overseas if you had WLS. I trusted SML's book in 2008 and I decided to trust her again. She got me through dumping my first time, she talked about how to deal with family and drinking and what to eat in her book. When I got here, I found out that so many people were in the same boat as me.

Regain. It's embarrassing. I felt like "I had an excuse — I had a baby". An excuse is like a butt...everyone has one. When do we let go of our excuses and really give our choices a once over — that's when we hit rock bottom.

I did that. I joined, I cried, and I listened. I whined, I complained and I justified. And then I pulled up my plus sized pants and got on the BOT train. I've lost 46 pounds since then, I'm stalled currently but I'm shooting to lose back to before my pregnancy and get down to a goal I never hit the first time around.

I'm telling you all my story because it's a cautionary tale of what happens when you start making excuses for bad choices. Babies are being born to WLS patients daily now and they are making better choices than I did. They are not gaining heaps of weight and justifying it for 4 years after. They are not finding themselves running for Mayor of Regainville.

I hope that each and everyone one of you embarking on the journey of Motherhood finds it as beautiful as I do. I also hope you don't make the same mistakes I did. Losing the second time around sucks.

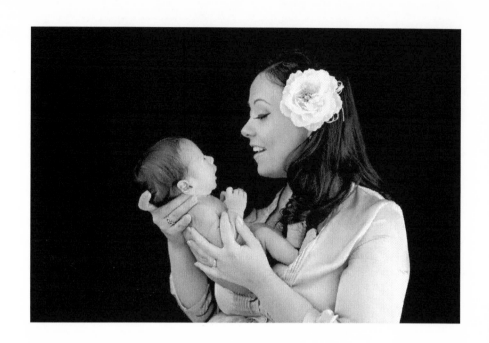

LIFE AFTER GASTRIC BYPASS - GOAL - REGAIN - LOSS AND LOVING MYSELF

"If You Don't Love Yourself, How In The Hell You Gonna Love Somebody Else?" – Rupaul

As a former plus size model and a global artist at Saks Fifth Avenue in NYC, I meet models and celebrities and just regular "thin" people daily. I worked with photographers who would complain that the light reflected off my cellulite or agencies who claimed I wasn't "plus size enough." I work on models who don't eat for three days before a shoot and their skin looks like it's about to fall off, yet they are labeled the most beautiful women alive. I often post personal photos and use Snapchat or Instagram filters to smooth out my wrinkles (hey, I am turning 36 next month) and I have no shame that I wear a full face of makeup daily. It's not about what I project out to the world as far as my appearance, it's my acceptance and pride in my appearance that shows through, regardless of size. It's always been like that for me.

At 402 pounds I could look into the mirror and feel beautiful. I didn't hate myself or my body. At 300 pounds I was in print magazines, on the walls of my favourite store and even one tiny billboard in LA.

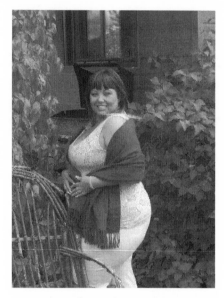

Kelsey in 2003

Beauty isn't about the number on the scale or the size on the tag of your pants. Beauty is so much more how you feel about yourself and thus what you radiate out into the world. But feeling beautiful at 400 pounds was going to kill me. Pride, even in my size 32 Lane Bryant pants, wasn't going to save me from heart disease, or diabetes. We are all here because medically we had a problem – and the weight loss needed professional help. Although my pride took a hit asking for that help – it saved my life. And believe me, I struggled to feel beautiful after WLS. I felt like a melting candle for awhile, unsure of how people would react to thinner legs that knees moved on their own like a Sharpei. I wasn't sure if I was "allowed" to feel good about my body since it had changed so much. Yes my weight was ALOT lower, but my body, it wasn't like those girls you see in magazines or on TV. I still looked different. And it took alot of self reflection, and alot of honesty to see that I was still beautiful, just a new style of beautiful! Plus seeing my body perform the miracle of pregnancy was absolutely INCREDIBLE! I've been up and down with regain and I'm finally back to where I was before I decided to have a baby.

But I'm struggling again now that I've lost all of my regain (98 pounds so far) I don't know where to end my loss because I could keep going. I look in the mirror today and I feel beautiful. I'm still obese class 2 — but my body looks good to me. Yes, I have loads of loose skin, and saggy bits. Yes, I'm not a size zero or wearing an extra small. But I feel good because I like being a bit on the curvy side. People at work exclaim how "tiny" I am — which is only in comparison to how I looked before I lost weight — not in relative terms to cover models or actually skinny people. My pants fit and I shop in regular clothing sections; my feet no longer hurt after 8 hours in heels, and I proudly wear a bikini to the pool, so am I done? Am I beautiful "enough" now?

Who gets to determine your beauty?

YOU!

It's not about a magazine telling us perfect proportions, or a music video showing the "thick" girls or even your boyfriend/girlfriend/husband/wife/partner/family/friend/etc. It's you. It's not about what plus size means or doesn't mean, or the normalization of skinny or fat.

I think it's time we celebrate the beauty in all forms – we here at BE are supporting your change for a healthier lifestyle, a better quality of life, and a path to help you see the beauty in yourself – but you need to look in the mirror and see it too.

I'm incredibly proud to have lost 256 pounds, and almost 98 a second time. I'm proud that Italian Vogue had the courage to show women who aren't size zero, and that Ashley Graham showed the world that the cover of Sports Illustrated isn't just for the ultra thin. But in reality, I hope each of those women feel beautiful in their own right and are not looking for justification from a society that just doesn't quite understand yet.

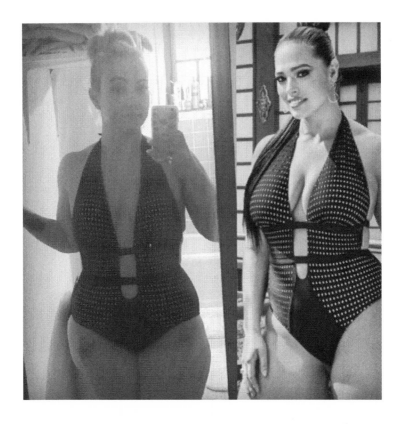

So I posted a picture a few weeks ago in response to a question about what everyone at around my height looks like after WLS. It kind of got me thinking as I scrolled through the photos. Who determines what the goal is, what your end weight should be? For me, I started off with a goal of 123. It was an easy number to remember 1-2-3 and my Doctor agreed for my height (4'11") it was a good goal. I realized when I got down to 146 and was miserable with how I looked -- that weight wasn't really my issue. It was my body image. I have a certain idea in my mind of how I like my body to look.

Now, I had RNY 10 years ago because I wanted to have a family. I wanted a baby so badly and this seemed like the only hurdle in my way. At 402 pounds, and after 6 miscarriages, my Doctor (who I hated at the time) finally said the words that cut deep -- you're just too heavy, your body is crushing your internal organs, how do you think a fetus will do in there?

I cried and cried and cried. And then I took a hard look in the mirror. Now, even at 402 pounds I wasn't ever ashamed of my body. I spent many years as a plus size model and I was even on a Billboard, my body image while I think looking back was skewed, but I felt good about me. Even when Lane Bryant pants could no longer fit. I still looked in the mirror happy with what I saw.

But my health. Anyway, I went on to lose 256 pounds. And when I got down to that 146 - I didn't like what I saw in the mirror and that was SO CONFUSING. I was supposed to be happy being thin. But the thing was, I wasn't losing weight because I hated how I looked, and this new body came so quickly, I had no idea what to do with it, how to dress it, why it wasn't firm anymore, why it hurt to run down the stairs, why my bras seemed weird, and I didn't recognize my own shadow.

Fast forward a few years, I maintained around 146-152 until I was FINALLY blessed with a successful pregnancy. After my little bones was born, I was up to 212. But I loved how my body looked. BUT I was in distress over the weight gain and terrified to get back up into the unhealthy weight I was before. It was a constant struggle of, oh I love how these pants fit, but I should be eating more salad. Being on a diet that my heart wasn't really in was so hard.

I finally found Susan Maria Leach (again, her book was my bible 10 years ago) through FB and found these groups and my life changed. But even after I lost my regain (twice) I find myself looking at my body like it belongs to someone else.

Finally after many talks, and tears, and frantic text messages to my bestie -- both her and our beloved Founder helped me to realize, maybe I was at goal. No it wasn't 146, it was around 175 and although my brain kept telling me to get to my lowest weight, my heart said, you love your body now and you're healthy -- what's the problem??

The moral of this LONG story is that only you get to determine where your end goal is. And that might change a few times over the course of your new life. I've learned how to dress this body that I'm in love with to suit my tastes and my ideals of beauty. I've learned to be comfortable in my own skin even if I'm not in a size 4 like before. It's not about numbers, it's about you and what you truly love about you.

Needless to say, I'm 36 and I live a really stressful hectic life. I'm never perfect as far as my diet and my weight fluctuates alot. But instead of relying on the number on my scale (although I do weigh myself a few times a month) I look in the mirror -- I notice how my clothes fit and I try to remember that the REASON I had WLS was to be a Mama, and my little bones (who is now 6) needs an active, healthy and happy Mama -- not one obsessed with numbers on a scale or how many calories are in veggies. So I treat my body in a way that will ensure I'm able to do all the things a Mama needs to do -- like run around the park, or carry sick 6 year olds to bed, or live long enough to see Grandbabies. I treat my body like my son's biggest protector and I feed it good things to keep me healthy. And that's what hitting a goal should feel like.

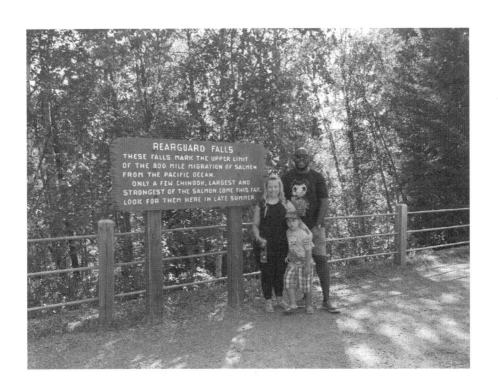

3500 CALORIES.

That is the amount that it takes to gain 1 pound. It doesn't matter if you're a body builder, have PCOS, live in Alaska or had overweight parents. The human body requires 3500 calories to make one pound.

One of the hardest hurdles to overcome when it comes to weight loss surgery is that if you don't let go of your excuses -- you'll never be able to attain long term success. The first 16 months make you feel invincible, like you're doing everything right even if you're not actually (like sneaking foods you know you shouldn't). What happens in the rest of your life, and the reason we have a massive group on Facebook of people who have had regain -- is the result of not identifying your excuses prior.

For me, it was that I was in control. I could have one tortilla a month because I had a craving. One became 4 which quickly spun out of control. But there are other deeply embedded excuses that we have a hard time letting go of.

One of these is the thought that you are genetically destined to be obese because your family has always been obese. Here is the thing: if you come from a typically obese family -- have a look at what you're eating and how much exercise you're getting. There is no obese family out there that is eating healthy lean protein meals with veggies on the side and fruit as dessert. We live in a time that counts on fast food as reliable sustenance for our families. We add cakes and pies and we have deep fryers at home. We rarely rely on the healthy lean meats and sprinkles of cheese and fresh fruit and instead we reach for dinner rolls, veggies cooked in copious amounts of butter or oil, and carb heavy main dishes.

Part of the problem is economic. It's cheap to eat highly processed carbs. But it's also laziness on our part. If eating healthy was really our MAIN concern, we'd find a way and create a budget and source out the fuel our bodies really need. Instead we take the easy way out -- yes I said it, and we consume the fast cheap stuff, complain about all that's going wrong in our bodies like we have no idea.

Morbid obesity and weight loss surgery are not the problem and solution. The problem is our mindset that we do not make healthy foods the only choice. The solution is just that.

And no one said it's going to be easy. In fact the hardest thing to learn is that your "reasons" are actually excuses and in order to be successful for the rest of your life, you have to own up to that. I made a list of my "reasons" that were actually excuses and it was incredible what I had convinced myself of. Imagine if I could use that super power to convince myself that I really wanted to be healthy and eat things to make my body strong instead of making it weak?

DATING AFTER WLS

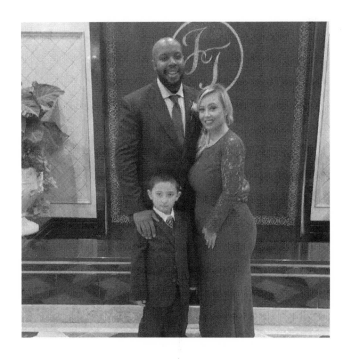

I wanted to touch on a topic that alot of post ops struggle with. Dating after Weight Loss Surgery.

So alot of us go through this journey, we lose weight, and we start to attract different attention than we did before.

Usually it's surprising and we are caught off guard. I have seen so many post op women struggle in bad relationships after losing their weight because they settle for the first person that comes along.

Let me back track a bit. What's your favourite colour? Mine is black - but that doesn't mean I don't like all the other colours, I just like black the best. Sexual attraction is sort of like that. Men and women come in all different shapes and sizes and because of that, everyone has their own "type" and that can include appearance. AND THAT IS OKAY.

I want to repeat -- that is okay. Remember my favourite colour, yellow can't get offended that I like black - I'm entitled to like whatever appeals to me.

Okay so bodies. Some men and women loved us when we were morbidly obese, maybe you're even married and your spouse is seeing a whole new you emerge and it's a completely different appearance than he or she fell in love with. I'll touch more on this later.

So you've got this hot new body and you're starting to get attention from new men and women. This feels really weird at first. I remember being so offended, like "wasn't I pretty to you before?" but the truth is, they prefer a body shape that looks more like my body does now. And again, THAT IS OKAY.

So you're getting all this new attention and you start dating... remember that even if you spent years alone, you are entitled to find your own type. You don't have to settle for the first person who comes along. Or maybe you meet the one and it's love at first sight. Either way, honour yourself first - like Rupal says, "aint nobody gonna love you if you don't love yourself".

So that being said... if you're single, get out there and mingle. A few things to keep in mind.

Drinking: be careful. Alcohol as a post op is a tricky tight rope. Alcohol hits us really hard after weight loss surgery and even the most seasoned drinker can have really adverse reactions. Be sure you have a full night game plan, and people you trust with your life (literally--not first date material) and be sure you've eaten beforehand. Stay clear of sugary drinks as they will make you very quickly sick, but a glass of wine or a cocktail in seltzer water is okay.

Secondly, you don't have to wear your WLS on your sleeve. There are no hard and fast rules about this, but you don't have to tell anyone. Did you know that regular slim people order salads regularly at restaurants? Or eat small portions? You don't have to answer for your dietary restrictions -- and a date is not the time to pull out your bariatric card for eating off the kids menu...

Thirdly, be choosey. I don't know how to say this without sounding crass so I'm going to say it like I'm your older sister. As former fat people who likely felt somewhat insecure about ourselves, it feels new and exciting to have someone want to take you out and maybe touch you. YOU DO NOT OWE anyone anything. If you don't want to kiss on the first date, you don't need it, you play by your own comfortable terms. End of story.

And lastly, I want to share a secret with you -- that loose skin that you're freaking out about someone seeing? They don't care. Bodies are really cool and the stretch marks and loose skin are never going to deter someone who cares about you -- so let that insecurity go. What's sexy? Being comfortable in your own skin. What's not sexy? Wanting to turn the lights off and acting weird about how your body looks. IF someone wants to be intimate with you, and you're willing, don't let a beautiful moment get all messed up over some skin.... trust me, they don't care.

I also want to talk to the married folks out there. I'm sure you've seen the stats, and how many marriages fall apart after weight loss surgery. This can happen for a myriad of reasons. The key to keeping a healthy and happy marriage after wls is communication. Talk to your spouse about how your body is changing, and how they feel. But remember it's your body and you get to determine what it looks like. Some spouses will have a very hard time with your new found attention and take it gracefully. I have found that most of the happy marriages that last through weight loss surgery are ones of open and honest communication.

On the flipside, I've encounter alot of people who settled and married someone they maybe shouldn't have because they didn't feel worthy of love and affection. And once they lose weight they realize that they are in fact worth more than the crappy relationship they are in. This is also okay. Life itself is a journey -- and some relationships are not meant to last forever.

So you're ready to start dating - but where is the best place to go? Online dating communities are really popular and mainstream now and I know alot of great couples who found each other that way. The gym and other healthy hobby places are a great spot to meet someone to share your new lifestyle. But the best way? Just be your confident amazing self everywhere you go. Confidence is sexy and everyone is attracted to that person who feels good about themselves.

So to recap some tips on dating after WLS:

1. Be careful drinking on dates
2. You don't have to tell anyone you had WLS.
3. Respect yourself and your body.

4. No one will notice or care about your loose skin.

5. Have fun and be confident!

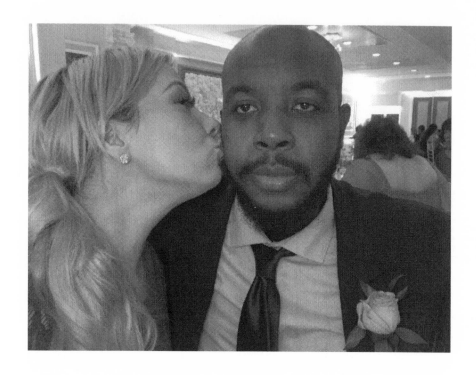

LOSING WEIGHT AND FRIENDSHIPS

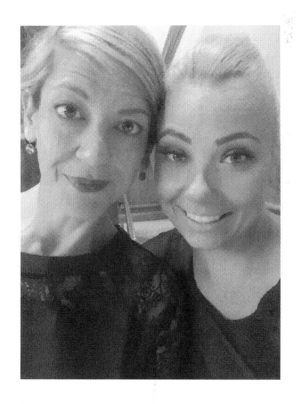

As human beings we are built to be incredibly social creatures. We enjoy meeting people and spending time with loved ones and friends. Often obesity runs hand in hand with this socializing nature. Going out to dinner and drinks or girls brunch on the weekends, or just grabbing a bite to eat with someone else fills that need to NOT be alone.

So what do you do when all of a sudden that's not the norm for you anymore. Going out to dinner at Chinese buffets isn't appealing and the late night cocktails don't fit your diet anymore -- do you lose your friends?

Sometimes yes and sometimes no. This really depends on what you deem important to you after your weight loss surgery. If you are someone who is struggling really hard with good food choices - likely going out to eat is going to be very difficult for you. If you are trying to give up alcohol - maybe the bar isn't a great hang out with friends. But what happens when we shy away from these activities to reset our new lives and all of a sudden our phone stops ringing with invitations?

First things first, it isn't you. You are making a great choice to respect yourself and your body and getting a handle on the first things that lead you to surgery for obesity is the first and best step. Secondly, it's not forever, sometimes we just need a little time to come to terms with this new lifestyle and then we can move on and re-enter our social circles stronger than before.

But it's painful when you're friends and family stop calling. You start feeling isolated and withdrawn and often angry and upset. Realize that "fair weather" friends aren't really worth your time. If someone only wants to hang out with you to eat crappy food -- what kind of a friend is that? If your friendship revolved around poor life decisions and now you're ready for your best life - you need people around you who share your same goals and ideals. You need people around you who will support you and help propel you further and not pull you down.

The same goes for family. Don't let anyone guilt you into "just one bite" of something that's not a part of your plan. Or guilt you into skipping the family BBQ because "everyone feels uncomfortable eating around you." You get to be the captain of your own ship - and you get to make the choices for yourself. Likely there wasn't anyone there suffering alongside you when your obesity became a surgical option - nor were they there when you were miserable and unhealthy so they don't get to dictate what you're going through now. You do, be firm. Eventually they will understand and come around.

Also what is really cool is that the new you might like new things! Like the gym or the park or any other healthy lifestyle activities. You are likely going to meet some new people who enjoy the same things you do and you'll make more friends. Life is a journey and it's always changing - you can go with the flow or you can be the flow - you choose.

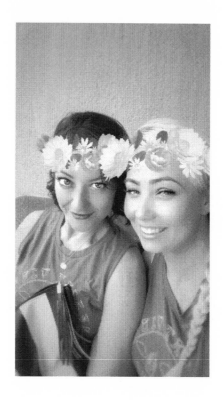

MY TOP TEN BARIATRIC TIPS

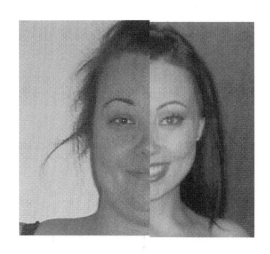

10. Nobody really understands unless they've had weight loss surgery too. And that's okay. But don't try to impose your new body, diet, lifestyle, etc onto them. They won't get it. And your feelings will get hurt and it will cause fights. Nobody needs to know why you're now choosing a salad over fries. This is your journey.

9. No matter how much you lose – this lifestyle is forever. Trying to jump back into a "old eating habits" is the fast lane

to regain. Follow the rules – for life.

8. If you like your teeth and your bones – take your vitamins. Most of my weight loss surgery friends have lost lots of teeth, broken bones, needed extra surgeries from vitamin deficiencies. And no – Flintstones don't count.

7. Everyone has the surgery for different reasons – but we all ate too much of the wrong stuff. Get over your "woe is me" reasons and embrace that you are here making a change. Obesity doesn't target those who have health, emotional, physical, and mental issues. We made the choice to eat what we did. Time to move on. Same goes for regain. Take responsibility and move on. Back on Track is your cheat sheet.

6. Your skin will never be the same. It will sag and pucker. We stretched it out being overweight enough to need weight loss surgery. It likely won't ever be back to Barbie consistency without surgical help. And guess what? That's your choice too. I look like a melted candle naked – but Spanx helps and I'd rather wear shape-wear and single digit sizes than double digit sizes and have "firm" skin.

5. Drink your water. My four hospitalizations for dehydration sucked. The terror when you have no idea what is wrong and you legitimately think you might be dying —

and its dehydration, can be avoided. Our bodies are made of water, you're shrinking, drink the liquid.

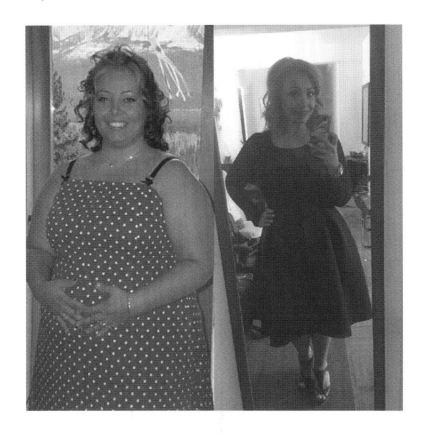

4. Find your own style. At 402 pounds: I wore what I thought looked good. Now I do the same. My body looks good in form fitting clothes — even though it may not be "on trend" or whatever. Find the fun in showing off your new figure! I still mainly wear black but now I've got heels on!

3. Celebrate yourself! This isn't easy by any means. It's actually really really hard. And it's not hard for a few months. It's hard FOREVER. So celebrate yourself and your

successes. Set goals and reward yourself (just make the rewards not food based for maximum awesomeness).

2. Protein powder is forever. You will never be able to eat enough protein to keep your body in prime condition. Find one you love (mine is clearly Inspire Peanut Butter Cookie – and this was after 8 years of trying every single other brand out there). Trust me – you need protein shakes forever.

1. Laugh at the cloud bread. Or the low carb tortillas. Or the million other substitutes out there trying to reel you in. They are NOT worth it. Find new foods to fall in love with. **Low carb tortillas took me to a 90 pound regain** – it's not worth the year of fighting to lose that regain. You can lose your regain but wouldn't it be even better to not have to? I can assure you the answer is yes.

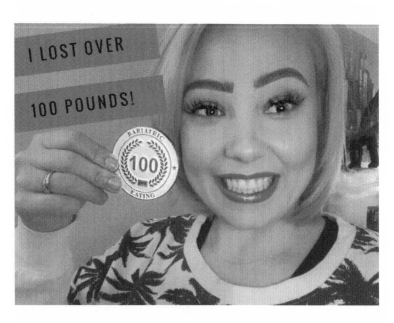

2007-TODAY!

So there you have it. My story, the ups and downs and all the in between. Sound familiar? I am one of millions of people around the world who have had weight loss surgery to create a better life for myself; BUT every single journey is different. Don't get too stuck on one hill in this adventure - the destination is ever changing, just like you. Thank you so very much for letting me tell you my story!

If you want to know more about me and learn more about WLS, Regain, Beauty and Fashion tips for Bariatric post ops please follow me on the following links:

❖ Facebook: http://www.facebook.com/wlsfinishingschool
❖ Instagram: http://www.instagram.com/wlsfinishingschool
❖ YouTube: http://www.youtube.com/bariatricbeautyfinishingschool

Here is the website if you're interested in The Inspire Diet to lose your Regain and the World's Best Bariatric Products Ever Made!

- ❖ http://www.bariatriceating.com -- for the World's Best Bariatric Products

Again, THANK YOU for being a part of my journey!
xoxoxo
Kelsey

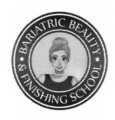

36614391R00043

Made in the USA
Columbia, SC
27 November 2018